Tara Binns
Big Idea Engineer

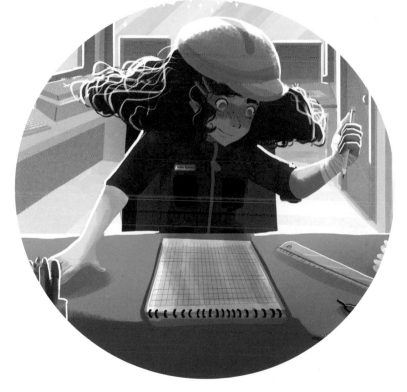

Written by Lisa Rajan

Illustrated by Alessia Trunfio

Collins

Chapter 1

There it was – dusty and a bit scratched, in the attic at the top of the house – the old costume box! Tara Binns grinned happily. She lifted the lid and her eyes shone as she looked inside.

The box was full of clothes, uniforms, shoes and hats. There was a costume for every job you could think of.

Every time Tara opened the box, it chose a different outfit for her … and sent her off on an exciting adventure.

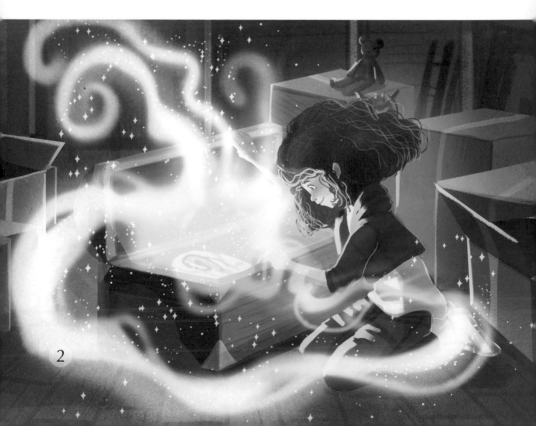

Her hands started to tingle … then the tingling spread up her arms … and around her whole body. A shining mist swirled up out of the box and whirled around her.

Suddenly, Tara found herself spinning and tumbling through space and time. She closed her eyes and wondered …
What will I be today?

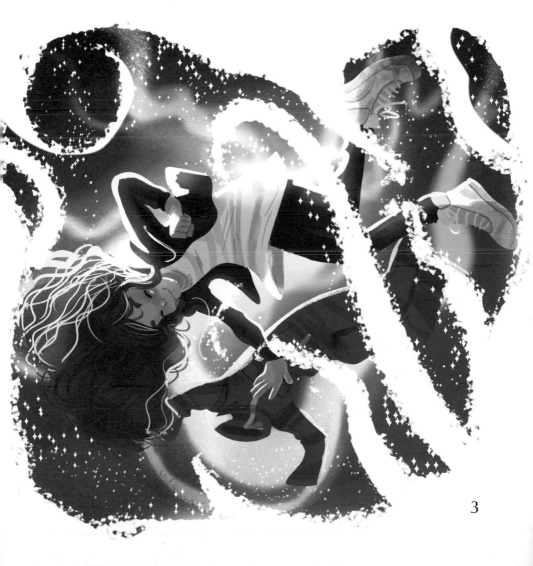

Chapter 2

The mist cleared and the world stopped spinning. Tara looked down at herself. She was wearing a white hard hat and navy overalls. There were safety goggles protecting her eyes. She was an engineer!

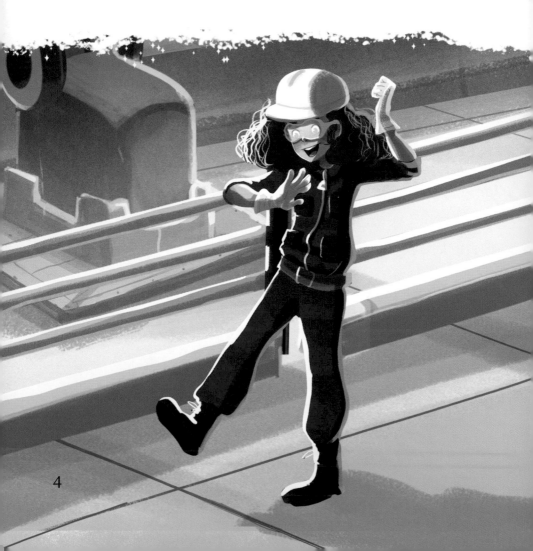

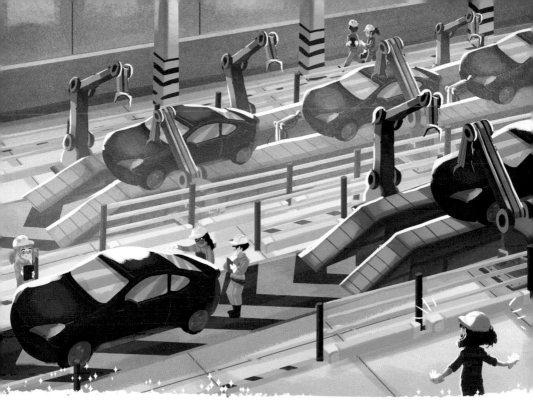

Tara was in a car factory. She could see the cars being built on the production lines. It was very noisy – motors running, machinery whirring and drills screaming.

In front of her, huge robots were fitting wheels on to a long line of cars. As each car was finished, an engineer checked it over, to make sure that it was perfect. Then the engineer hopped in the car and drove it away.

Tara heard the noise of an engine behind her. Wait … where was *that* car going? And why was it going so fast?

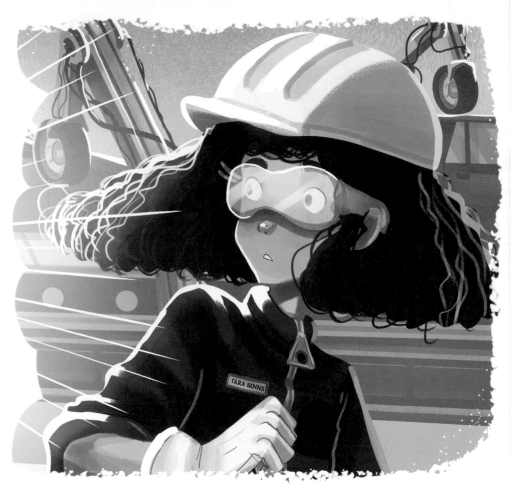

Tara watched the car speeding across the factory floor.
Luckily, there was no machinery there, just a big empty
space. But what was that? Oh! There was a concrete wall
at the far end, and the car was hurtling towards it at top
speed. Tara couldn't believe her eyes! Why wasn't the driver
slowing down? The car seemed to be speeding up … going
faster and faster! It was going to hit the wall!

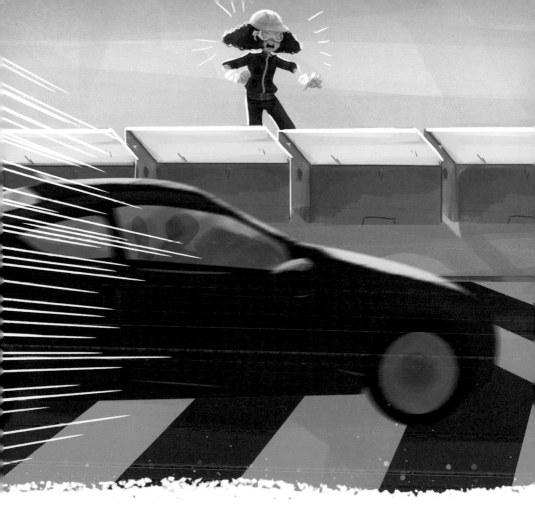

Something must be wrong with the car! Or maybe something had happened to the driver? Maybe he was ill … maybe he'd fainted.

"Hey!" she shouted. "*STOP!* You're going to CRA—"

SMASH!

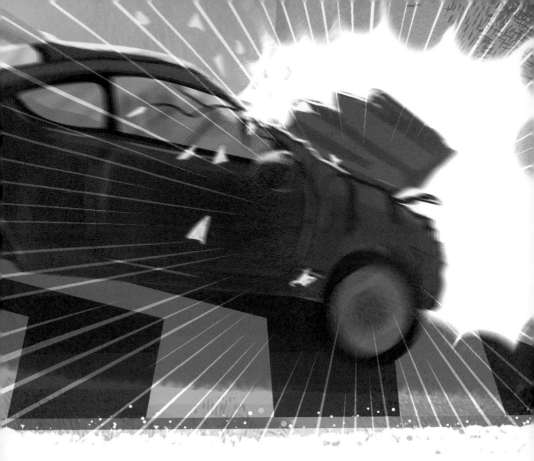

The car slammed headlong into the wall.

A huge BANG echoed all over the factory. Tara clapped her hands over her ears.

The front of the car crumpled instantly. Bits of plastic flew in all directions. The windscreen and the windows were smashed.

Oh no – what a terrible crash! Tara had never seen a car so badly smashed.

The driver! He or she must be hurt. I must help – and quickly, she thought.

Tara raced towards the car. But in her panic, she didn't look where she was going.

OOOPS!

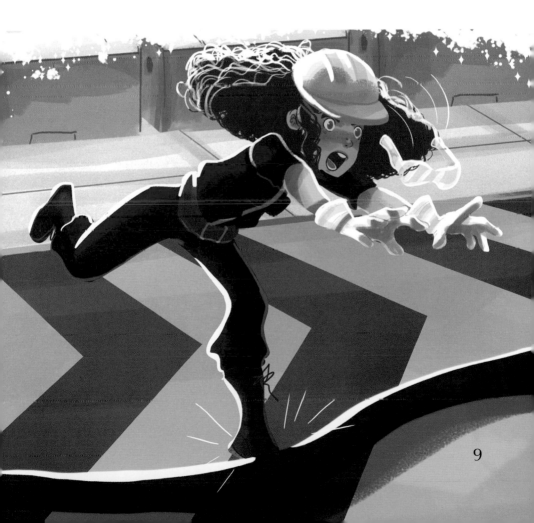

Chapter 3

Tara tripped over a thick black cable snaking across the floor. She went flying forward.

AAARGH!

She crash-landed on her hands and knees. The concrete floor was rock hard.

OUCH! That hurt!

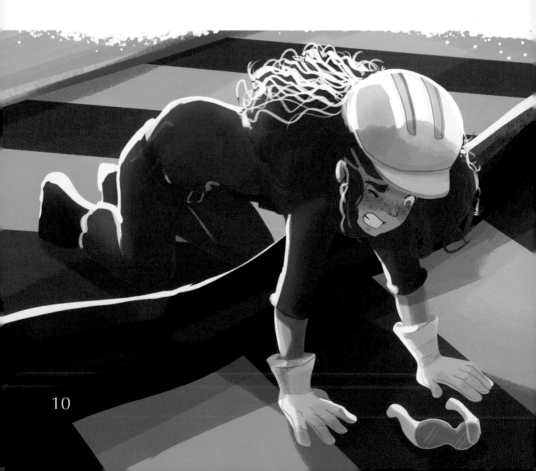

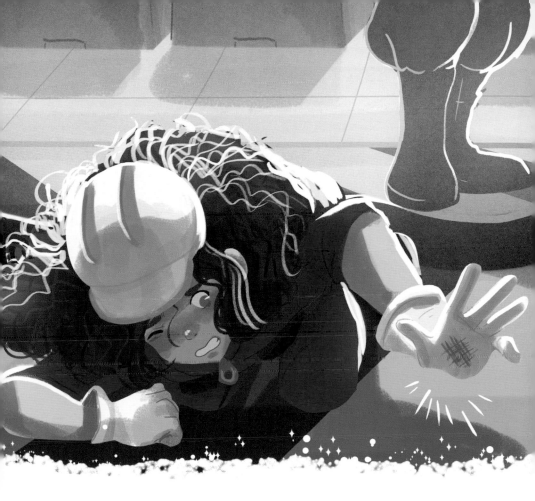

Tara lay there, sprawled on the floor for a moment. Pain shot through her knees and hands. Tears sprang to her eyes.

Slowly, she put her hands flat on the floor and tried to push herself up. *Ow!* It was painful.

"Are you all right?" came a worried voice from behind her.

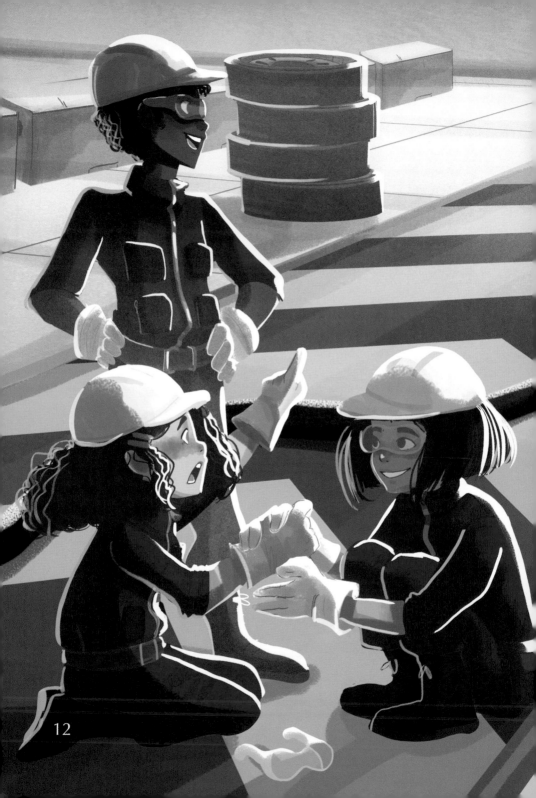

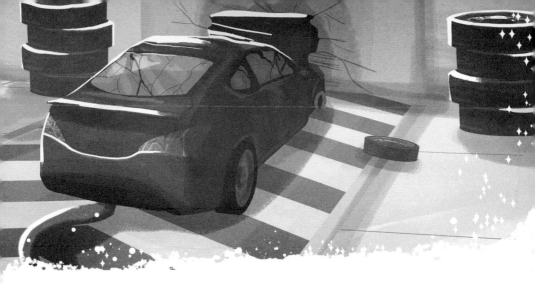

"That was quite a fall," the girl spoke again. "Let us help you. I'm Ayesha and this is Ortez. We're the chief safety engineers today."

Ayesha helped Tara to sit up.

"Sit there and rest for a moment," Ayesha went on. "We'll fetch the first-aid kit. Where are you hurt? Your knees? I'm not surprised. We saw you fall over. That was quite a bang!"

"Yes, my knees are hurting, and my wrist. But you shouldn't be worried about me! What about the driver of that car?" Tara spluttered.

"Kristoff, you mean?" said Ortez, looking at the smashed car. "Don't worry about him. He'll be fine. He always is!"

"What do you mean?" demanded Tara.

Ayesha smiled.

"Kristoff is a crash test dummy. He's used to smashing into that wall. We do controlled crashes like this every week. Come and meet him."

Ortez helped Tara walk to the car. He opened the driver's door.

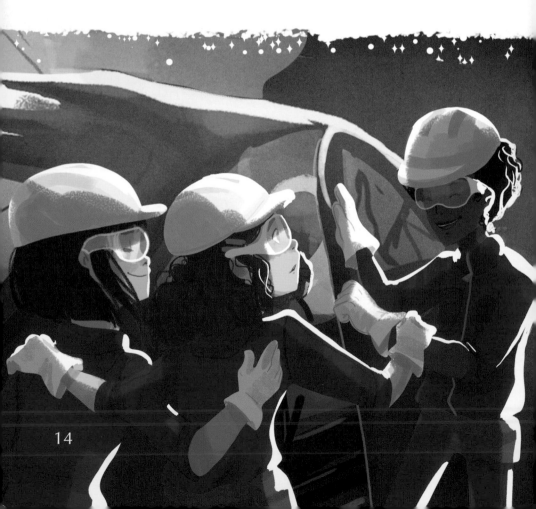

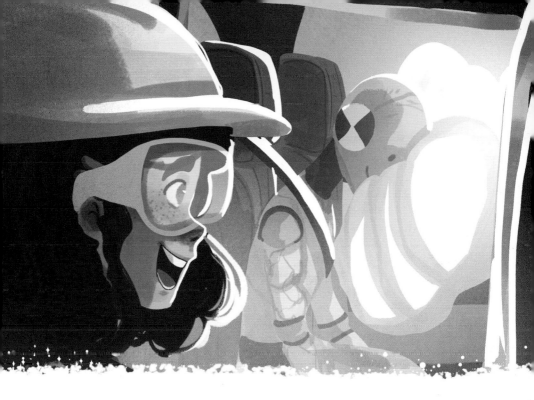

Sure enough, there was a plastic dummy behind the wheel.

"He's all right!" cried Tara. "Wow, I thought he'd have a big bump on his head after that smash!"

"Saved by the airbag," said Ortez. "Sensors on the car tell the airbag when the car hits something. The airbag inflates quickly and makes a cushion between the driver and the steering wheel. It stops the driver getting hurt."

"Lucky Kristoff!" said Tara.

Ayesha pulled Kristoff out of the driver's seat. His legs were bent and scratched. One of his arms had a huge dent in it. Maybe he wasn't so lucky after all.

"I know he looks a bit bashed up," said Ayesha, "but he helps us make cars safer. Engineers like us design cars to keep the driver and passengers safe. The best way to find out if our ideas work is to test them in a crash. But we can't use a real driver – it's too dangerous – so Kristoff steps up."

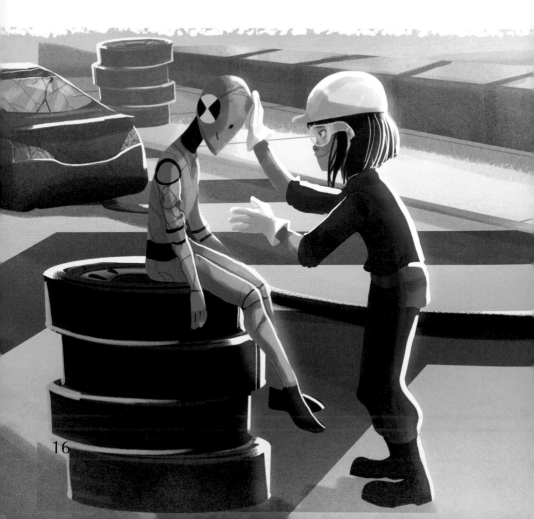

"Engineering is about solving problems, fixing things and improving them," added Ortez. "It's the perfect job for anyone with ideas and a keen imagination – and one eye on health and safety, of course! Here's the first-aid kit, if you need it."

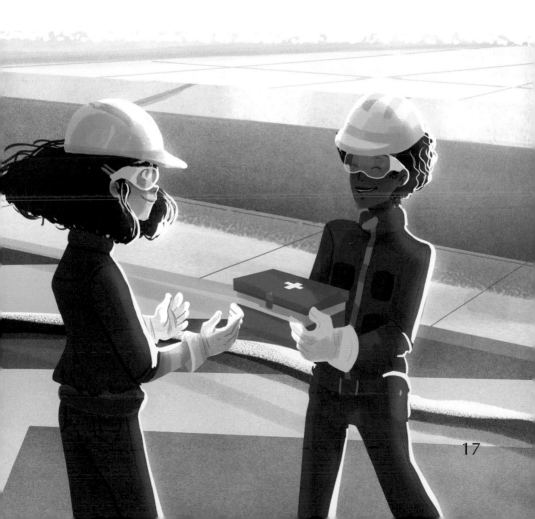

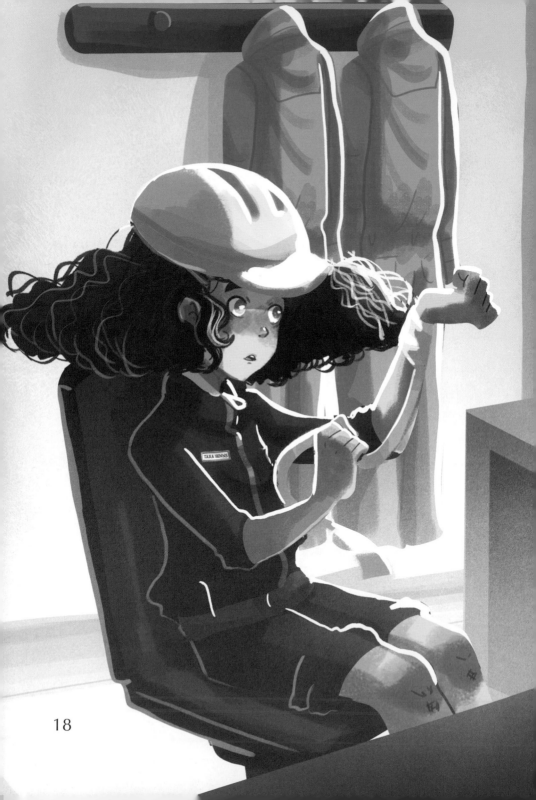

Chapter 4

Ortez and Ayesha went to examine the crashed car.

Tara sat down at their desk. She took a bandage from the first-aid kit. She wound it gently around her wrist.

My knees are still hurting, she said to herself. *I'll have massive bruises tomorrow. I hit the ground so hard and fast. I wish I'd had something to cushion the fall – like an airbag! If I'd had airbags in my trousers, then I wouldn't have hurt myself. Imagine …*

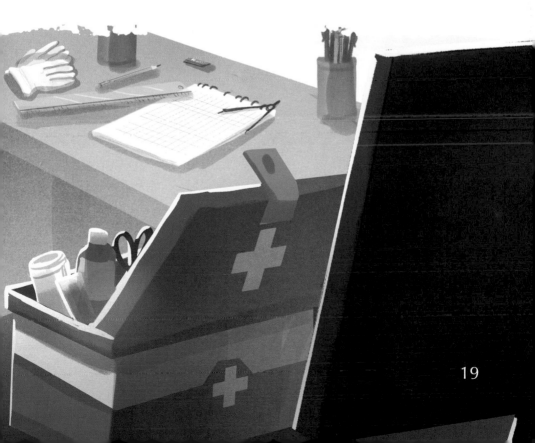

Tara began thinking.

Trousers that inflate when you hit the ground …

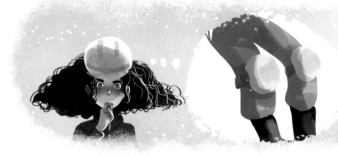

Maybe a whole suit that fills with air …

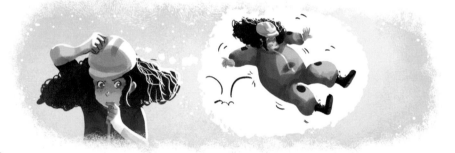

Gloves too, to protect your hands …

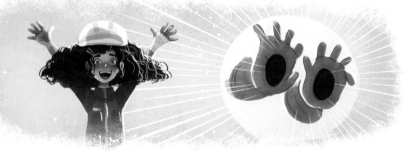

Wouldn't that be a clever idea?

What had Ortez said about engineers solving problems?
This could be the solution … clothes that puff up with air
if you are about to fall. It would be like having your own
personal airbag. The airbag would protect you if you fell on
a hard floor. The rest of the time it would secretly fold away,
so no one would know it was there.

I need a pencil and sketch pad, Tara thought. *I've got
to get this down on paper. I've just solved my first
engineering problem!*

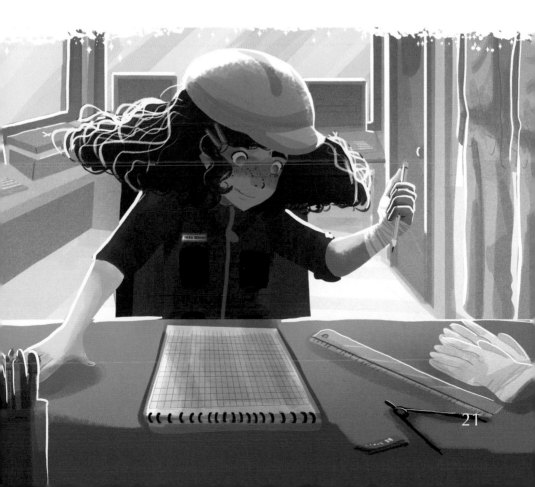

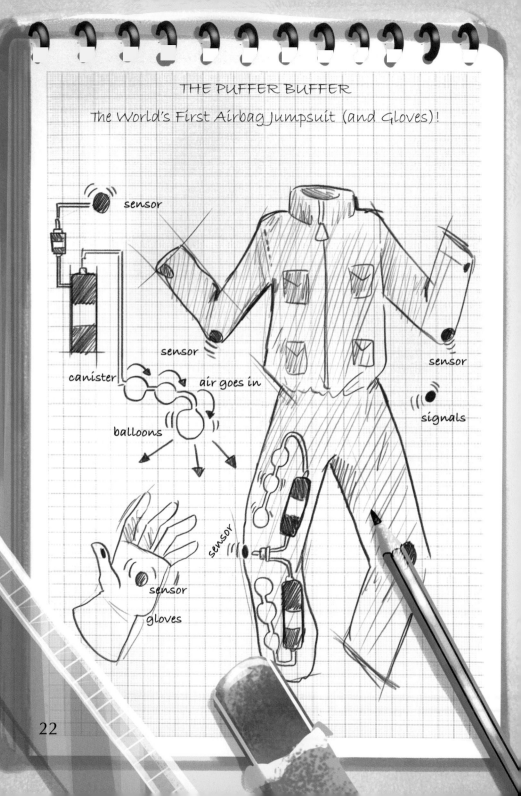

Tara found a sketch pad on the desk. She grabbed a pencil and began scribbling.

She drew, she sketched, she made notes.

She tweaked a bit here, she added a bit there.

She made the tubes longer and linked the balloons together.

She added sensors, which could tell if you were falling.

She added labels and arrows.

The finished sketch looked amazing. At the top, Tara wrote:

THE PUFFER BUFFER

The World's First Airbag Jumpsuit (and Gloves)!

On paper, her invention looked brilliant. But would it work?

Tara needed a second opinion. And a third.

"Ayesha! Ortez! Come and see my new invention," Tara called out to them. "I've just designed it!"

Ayesha and Ortez went over to the desk.

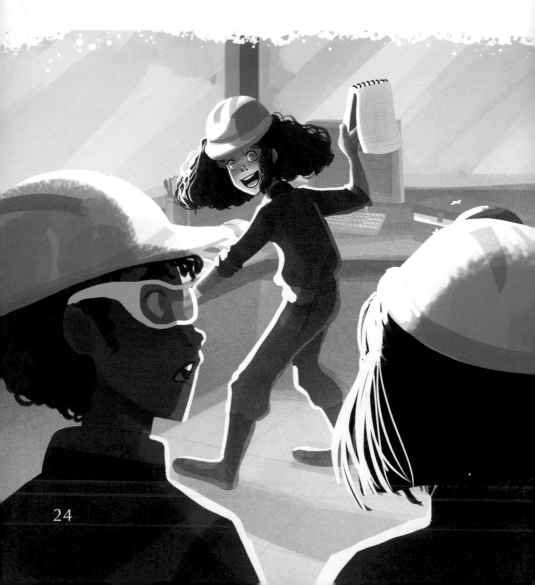

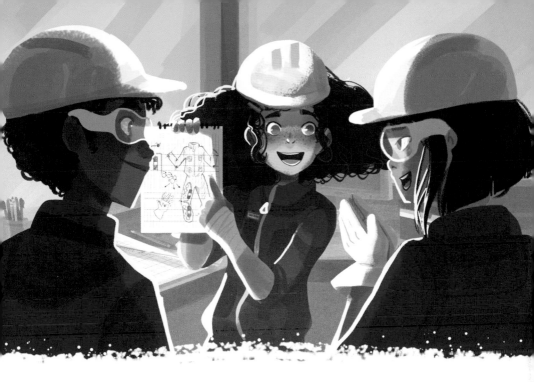

Tara talked them through her sketch.

"The sensors on the hands, knees and elbows are triggered when you fall. They send a message through these wires to these mini air canisters. The canisters blast air into the tubes – here. This inflates a string of mini airbags, like balloons, up and down the trouser leg – or around your elbow – there. Or on your hands – there. The whole suit becomes an airbag in less than a second. What do you think?"

"I think it's a fantastic idea!" said Ayesha. "Let's make one – right now!"

Chapter 5

Before long, the Puffer Buffer was finished. Tara pulled it on and zipped it up.

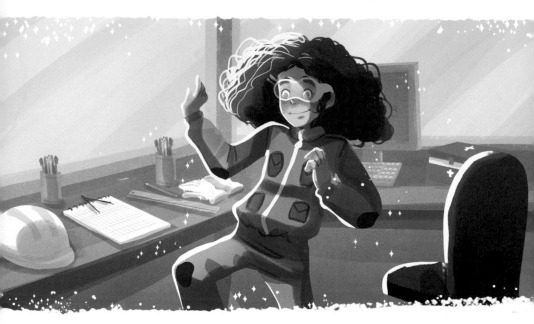

"It's lucky we had that spare pale blue suit. *Mm …* it fits perfectly."

She slid a hand into each glove. It felt very comfortable – she couldn't even tell the wires and tubes were there.

"I really want to know if it works," began Tara, "but I'd rather not try it out myself. My knees couldn't take another crash test."

"No," said Ayesha kindly. "No one should try out a new idea by themselves. It's much too dangerous. But I do know someone who can help us."

"Kristoff?" asked Tara.

"No, not Kristoff. He's already damaged. But one of his brothers or sisters will happily step in. Especially if it protects their arms and legs. Let's go and fetch another crash dummy. We'll put this airbag jumpsuit of yours to the test, Engineer Binns!"

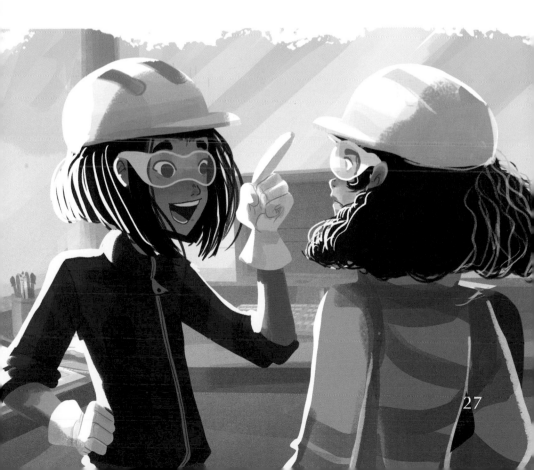

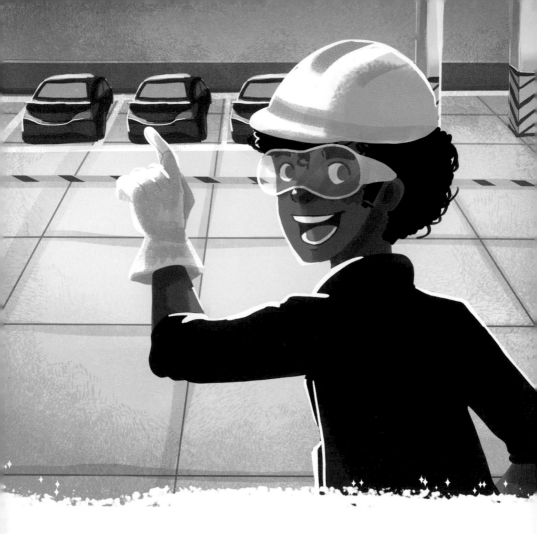

"I'll go and get another car," said Ortez, heading towards
the parking bays at the end of the crash test area.
"That's handy. Someone has just delivered three more cars.
They weren't here a minute ago."

Ayesha led Tara past the car production lines.

One of the lines had stopped working and the robots were still and quiet. An engineer was pointing at some oily droplets under one of the cars. He dipped a finger in the pale yellow liquid, rubbed it against his thumb, and sniffed it.

"Smells fishy," he said.

Tara frowned. "Does he mean something strange is going on?" she asked Ayesha.

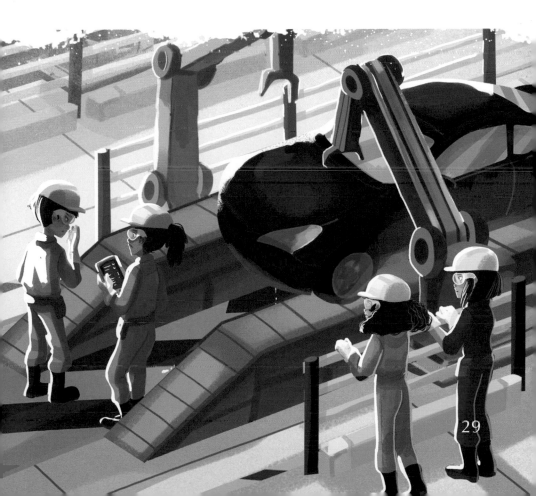

Ayesha explained. "No. He means it *actually* has a fishy smell. That means it's brake fluid."

Tara's eyes widened.

Ayesha went on, "When you want to slow a car down, you press the brake pedal, right? This pushes brake fluid into a thin pipe that runs along the underside of the car to the wheel. Look, I'll show you."

They both bent over and squinted up behind the wheel. It was difficult to see.

"The force of the brake fluid then pushes against brake pads that clamp either side of the brake disc in the wheel. This slows the wheel down and the car stops. If there's a hole in the pipe, the brake fluid runs out. The brakes won't work."

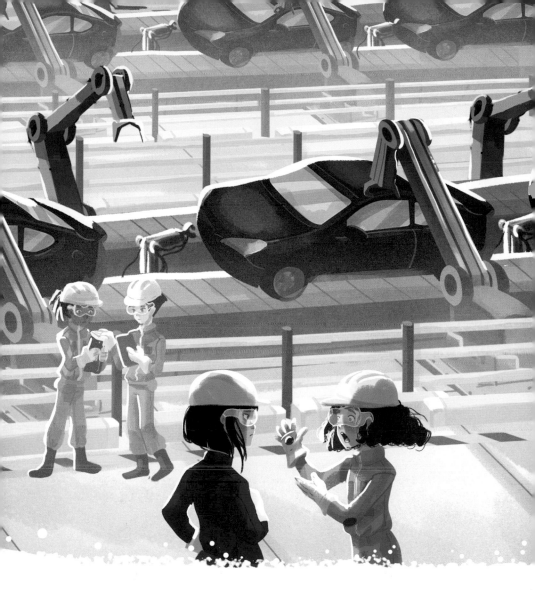

"But there's a hole in the brake fluid pipe before these cars have even left the production line," said Tara. "So it's worse than fishy. These cars are dangerous!"

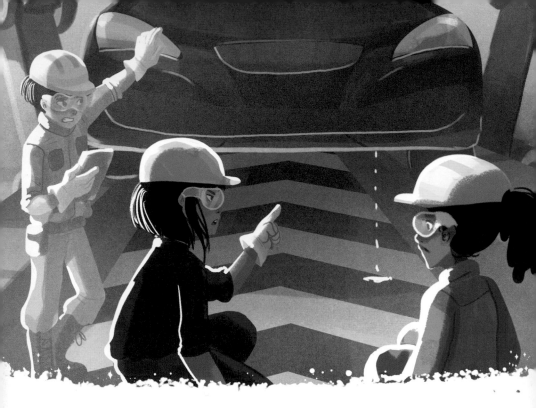

The engineers were looking under the car. Sure enough, there was a steady drip of oily, yellow fluid coming from the underside. Ayesha took a closer look.

"Brake fluid is leaking out of the pipe, all right," she said. "It looks like something has pinched it and made it split. I wonder why?"

The foreman looked worried.

"We've got to find out why," he snapped, "and quickly, or this production line will be held up!"

Tara's gaze followed the line of oily drips. They led towards the robot that worked on the underside of the cars. Her eyes narrowed. Was that—? Was that yellow brake fluid dripping off one of its pincer claws?

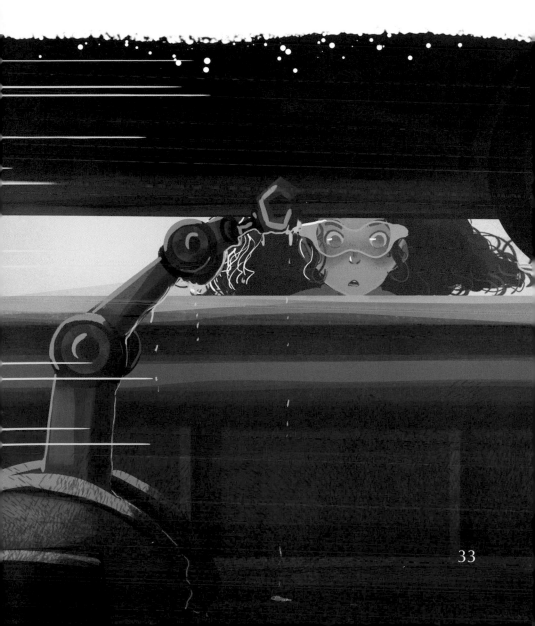

Chapter 6

"Look!" shouted Tara, pointing at the robot. "The claw of that robot has brake fluid on it. I bet that robot is splitting the brake pipe!"

Ayesha nodded. "Looks that way. We'll get an engineer to the production line to fix the robot as fast as possible."

Ayesha went to talk to the foreman about the robot.

Tara heard one of the engineers tell another to tow away the faulty car.

"Take it to the crash test area. The other three cars with faulty brakes are there already. We'll keep them safe until their brakes can be fixed. There aren't any more crash tests today, so they won't be a danger to anyone."

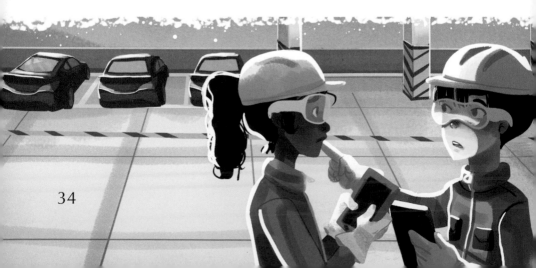

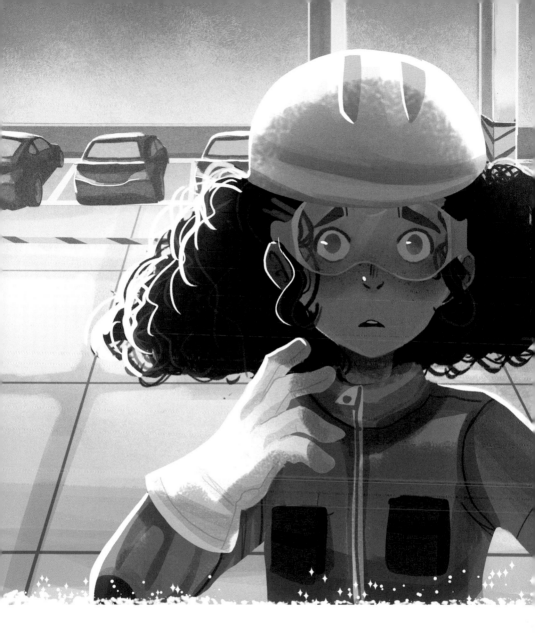

Tara was horrified. Ortez! He'd gone to fetch one of those faulty cars. He was about to drive a car with no brakes!

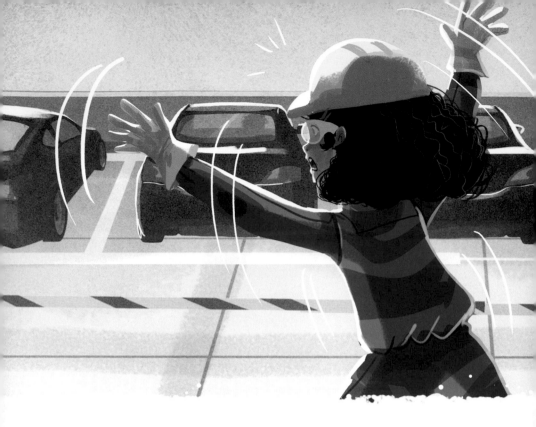

Tara had to do something quickly.

"ORTEZ!" she shouted. *"ORTEZ! STOP!"*

She could see him in the middle car.

"He can't hear me over the noise of the machinery," Tara realised. "I've got to warn him!"

She started running towards the car with faulty brakes, as fast as she could. *"ORTEZ! THAT CAR HAS NO BR—"*

She didn't see the pool of pale yellow brake fluid until it was too late.

WHOOPS!

For the second time that morning, Tara went flying through the air. And then she started falling …

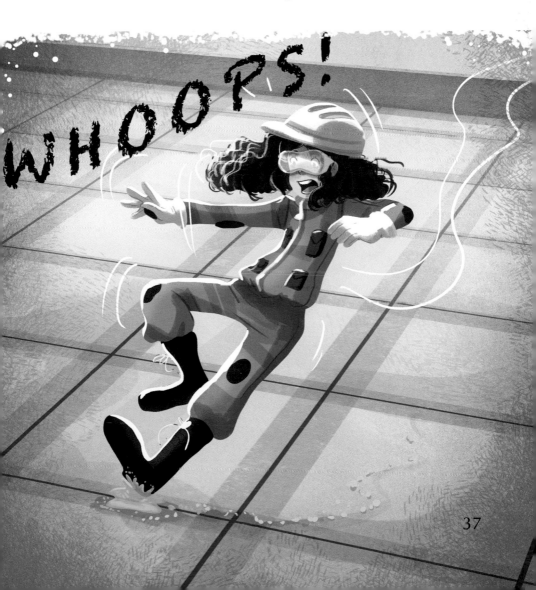

But in the split second before she hit the concrete floor, the sensors in her Puffer Buffer jumpsuit kicked into action.

They triggered the airbags … and *WHOOSH!* the Puffer Buffer inflated. Tara's knees landed on a soft cushion of air. She bounced! Twice! It was like being inside a balloon, protected by air on every side.

She rolled towards Ortez. At least, she thought she was heading in his direction. It was hard to know which way was up.

She heard the car door open.

"Tara! What are you doing?"

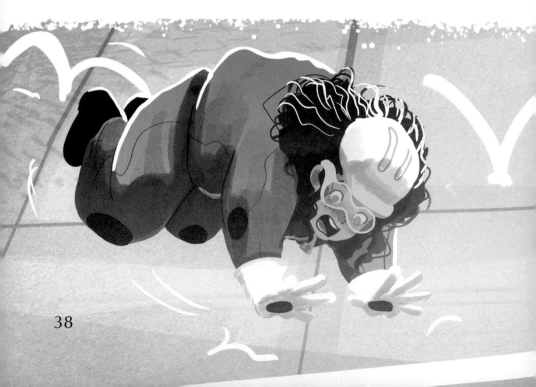

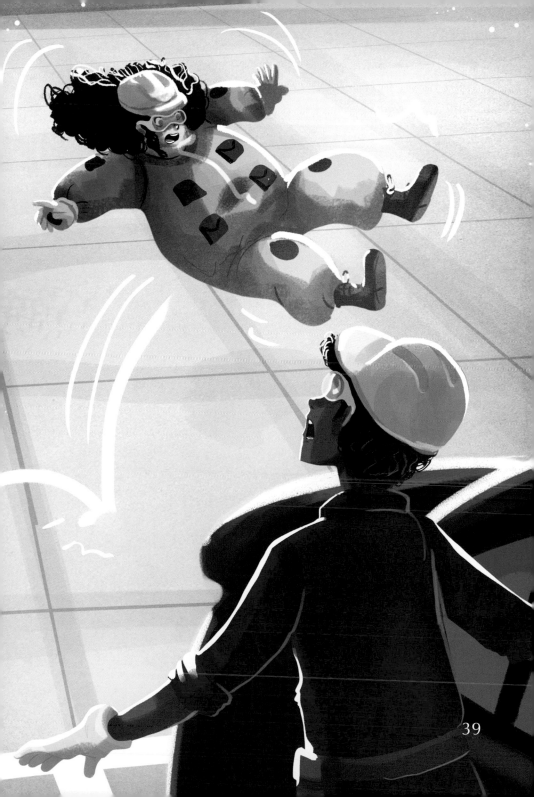

Chapter 7

Tara's jumpsuit started to deflate and she came to a halt. Ortez helped her to her feet.

"Thank goodness you didn't drive that car!" Tara said. "The brakes don't work! You would have crashed. I was coming to warn you but I slipped!"

"I was about to drive off, but then I saw a big blue beach ball bouncing around behind me," Ortez smiled. "I couldn't work out what it was. You stopped me just in time. Thanks, Tara – your invention saved both of us from getting hurt."

He looked serious. "But why was a car with faulty brakes parked in the test area?"

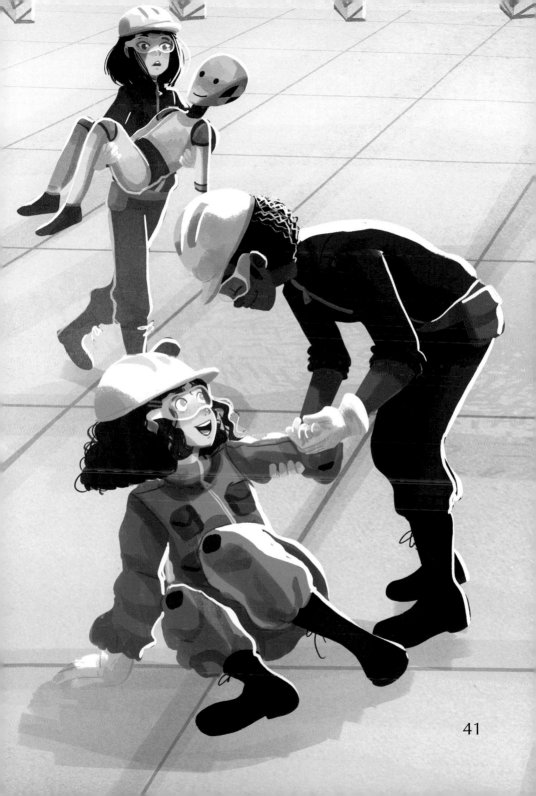

"There will have to be an investigation," agreed Ayesha, who had just arrived carrying a new crash test dummy.

"But Tara's invention worked," grinned Ortez. "She didn't hurt herself this time."

Ayesha looked pleased.

"Tara, your Puffer Buffer jumpsuit is amazing! Kristoff II is going to love it!"

Tara laughed.

"Now he can do all kinds of other safety test work – motorbikes, racing cars. He might even become a stunt dummy!"

"The sky's the limit," smiled Ayesha, "and for you too, Engineer Binns!" She raised her hand for a high five.

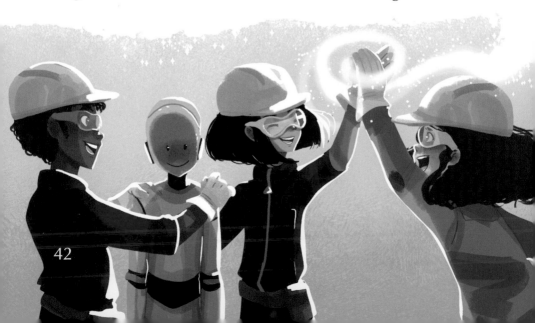

As Tara clapped her hand against Ayesha's, it started tingling. The tingling feeling travelled up her arm and all around her body. The factory started spinning ... or was it her? The cars ... the robots ... everything was whirling and swirling around her ...

KA-BOOM!

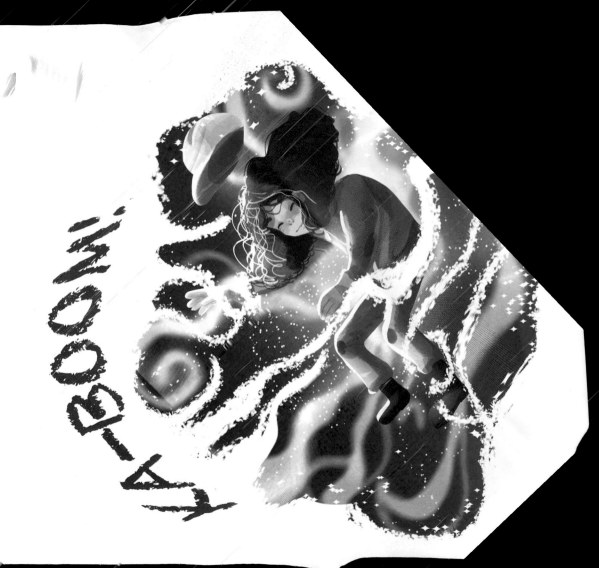

Chapter 8

The next moment, the world stopped spinning and Tara was back home in her attic.

She unzipped her engineer's overalls. She put the hard hat back in the chest. What an adventure to be an engineer and invent things! She loved having a big idea and showing that it could really work.

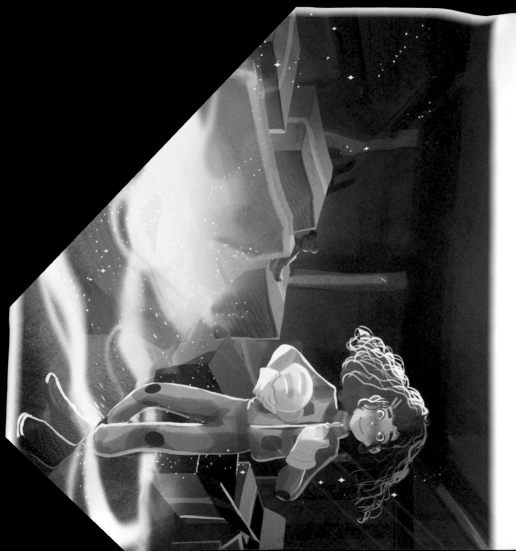

As Tara clapped her hand against Ayesha's, it started tingling. The tingling feeling travelled up her arm and all around her body. The factory started spinning … or was it her? The cars … the robots … everything was whirling and swirling around her …

KA-BOOM!

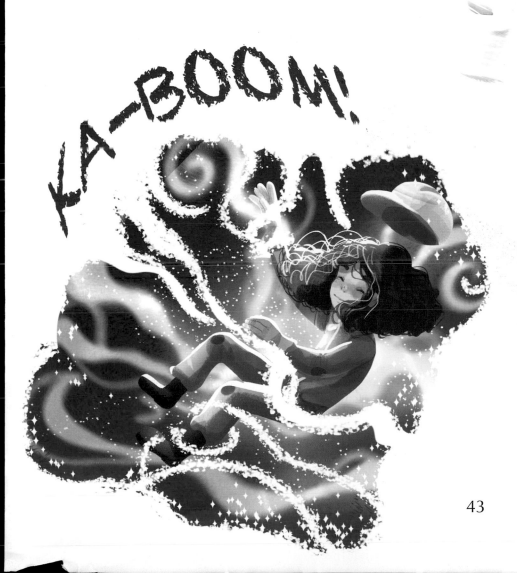

Chapter 8

The next moment, the world stopped spinning and Tara was back home in her attic.

She unzipped her engineer's overalls. She put the hard hat back in the chest. What an adventure to be an engineer and invent things! She loved having a big idea and showing that it could really work.

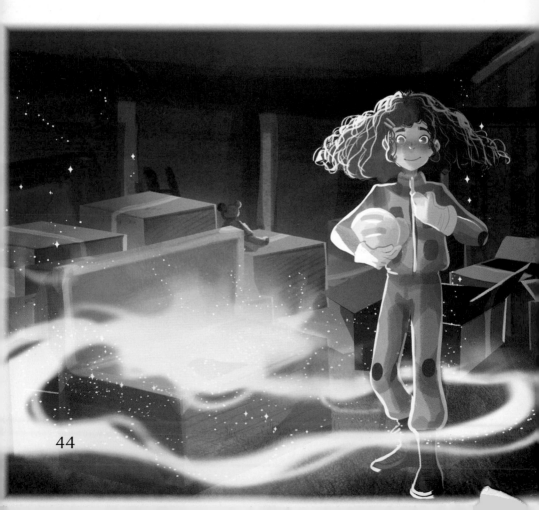

Tara closed the lid of the box and thought …

Maybe I'll be an engineer when I grow up. I'll have ideas, solve problems and fill the world with my new inventions!

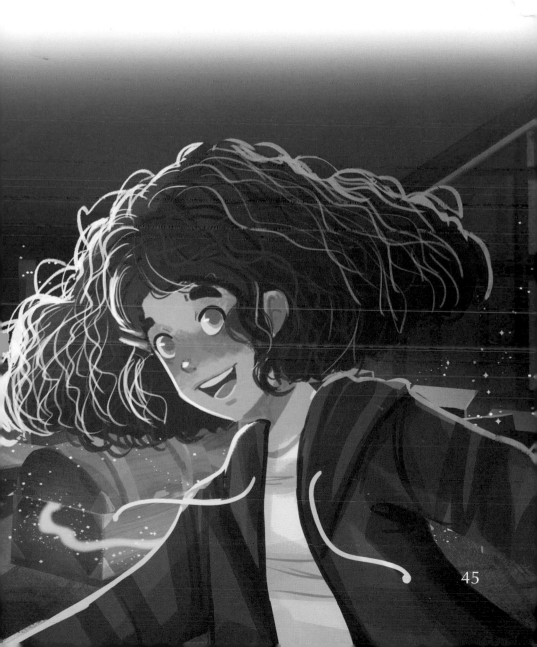

How does Tara Binns solve problems?

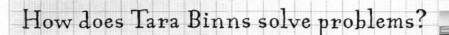

Falling over

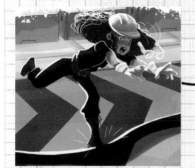 →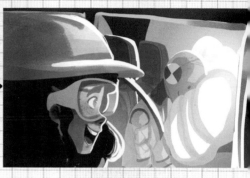

The brakes don't work

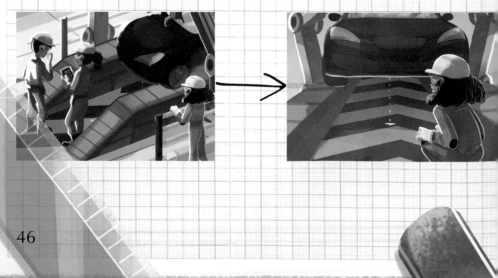